FIT FOR LIFE

A Comprehensive Guide to Health, Fitness, and Dieting

JAMES MAXWELL

This book is designed to provide general information on the subject of health, fitness, and dieting. It is not intended to be a substitute for professional medical advice, diagnosis, or treatment. Always seek the advice of your physician or other qualified healthcare provider with any questions you may have regarding a medical condition.

Thank you for respecting the hard work of the author and publisher.

TABLE OF CONTENTS

INTRODUCTION

The introduction of "Fit for Life: A Comprehensive Guide to Health, Fitness, and Dieting" sets the stage for the book by explaining why health, fitness, and dieting are important and how they are interconnected. It highlights the current state of health in modern society and the benefits of adopting a healthy lifestyle.

In our fast-paced and sedentary lifestyles, it is becoming increasingly important to take care of our health. Poor diet, lack of exercise, and stress can lead to a host of health problems such as obesity, heart disease, and diabetes. The good news is that making positive changes to our health, fitness, and diet can significantly reduce the risk of these and other health issues.

The purpose of this book is to provide a comprehensive guide to help you achieve optimal health and wellness through proper nutrition, exercise, and stress management. By following the advice and recommendations presented in this book, you can unlock your body's potential and achieve your health and fitness goals.

Whether you are looking to lose weight, build muscle, or simply improve your overall health, this book has something for you. The information presented here is backed by scientific research and practical experience, and it is designed to be easy to understand and apply in your daily life.

So, if you are ready to take control of your health and transform your life, read on!

Why Health, Fitness, and Dieting Matter

In the first section of "Fit for Life: A Comprehensive Guide to Health, Fitness, and Dieting", the book explores why health, fitness, and dieting matter. It delves into the benefits of leading a healthy lifestyle, the consequences of neglecting one's health, and the importance of adopting a holistic approach to wellness.

Understanding Your Body's Needs, introduces the concept of the human body as a complex machine that requires proper care and maintenance to function optimally. It discusses the basics of human anatomy and physiology, and how different systems in the body work together to maintain homeostasis. It also highlights the importance of listening to your body and paying attention to its signals.

The Importance of Sleep discusses the role of sleep in maintaining good health, both physical and mental. It covers the science of sleep, the benefits of good quality sleep, and the consequences of sleep deprivation. It also provides tips on how to improve sleep quality and establish healthy sleep habits.

Stress Management for Better Health This chapter explores the effects of stress on the body and mind, and how chronic stress can lead to a host of health problems. It provides strategies for managing stress, such as mindfulness meditation, yoga, and deep breathing exercises. It also discusses the importance of self-care and relaxation in reducing stress levels.

Overall, this section aims to provide readers with a foundational understanding of why health, fitness, and dieting matter. By understanding the importance of these aspects of wellness, readers can be motivated to take the necessary steps to improve their health and quality of life.

Part 1: Health Basics

Chapter 1: Understanding Your Body's Needs

In Part 1 of "Fit for Life: A Comprehensive Guide to Health, Fitness, and Dieting", the book focuses on the basics of health. It covers the fundamentals of how to take care of your body, including proper nutrition, hydration, and self-care.

This chapter introduces readers to the basic nutritional needs of the body, including macronutrients (carbohydrates, proteins, and fats) and micronutrients (vitamins and minerals). It also discusses the importance of hydration and provides tips on how to stay properly hydrated.

Your body is an incredible machine that requires proper care and maintenance to function at its best. In this chapter, we will explore the basic needs of your body, including water, nutrients, and oxygen, and how to meet them.

We will also discuss the importance of understanding your body's unique needs and how to listen to its signals. By the end of this chapter, you will have a better understanding of how your body works and what it needs to stay healthy.

Topics Covered:

- The Basics: Water, Nutrients, and Oxygen

- Understanding Your Body's Unique Needs

- Listening to Your Body's Signals

- Common Nutrient Deficiencies and How to Avoid Them

Whether you are just starting your health and fitness journey or looking to fine-tune your existing habits, this chapter will provide you with the knowledge and tools to make informed decisions about your body's needs.

Your body is a complex system that requires a variety of resources to function properly. From water to nutrients and oxygen, each component is vital to your health and well-being. In this chapter, we will explore the basics of your body's needs and how to meet them effectively.

The Basics: Water, Nutrients, and Oxygen

Water is essential for life. It makes up over 60% of your body and is involved in almost every bodily function, from digestion to temperature regulation. Dehydration can cause a range of health issues, from headaches and fatigue to more serious conditions like kidney stones and heatstroke. It's important to drink enough water throughout the day to maintain optimal hydration levels.

Nutrients are the building blocks of your body. They provide energy, support growth and repair, and keep your immune system functioning properly. Macronutrients, including carbohydrates, proteins, and fats, are needed in larger quantities, while micronutrients, like vitamins and minerals, are required in smaller amounts. A well-balanced diet that includes a variety of nutrient-rich foods is crucial to meeting your body's nutritional needs.

Oxygen is necessary for cellular respiration, the process by which your body produces energy. Your lungs take in oxygen with each breath, and it is transported to your cells via your bloodstream. If your body is not getting enough oxygen, you may experience symptoms like shortness of breath and fatigue.

Understanding Your Body's Unique Needs

While your body has basic needs that must be met, the exact requirements can vary from person to person. Factors like age, gender, activity level, and health status can all impact your body's needs. It's important to take a personalized approach to your health and wellness by understanding your body's unique needs and tailoring your habits accordingly.

Listening to Your Body's Signals

Your body is constantly sending you signals about its needs. Hunger, thirst, fatigue, and pain are all examples of signals that your body may be sending. It's important to pay attention to these signals and respond appropriately to prevent issues like dehydration, malnutrition, and injury.

Common Nutrient Deficiencies and How to Avoid Them

Many people do not get enough of certain nutrients in their diets. Common nutrient deficiencies include iron, vitamin D, and calcium. It's important to identify potential deficiencies and take steps to prevent them, such as increasing your intake of nutrient-rich foods or taking supplements.

By understanding your body's needs, you can make informed decisions about your health and wellness. In the following chapters, we will explore strategies for meeting your body's needs through diet, exercise, and lifestyle habits.

CHAPTER TWO

The Importance of Sleep

In Chapter 2 of "Fit for Life: A Comprehensive Guide to Health, Fitness, and Dieting", the book focuses on the importance of sleep for overall health and well-being. It covers the science of sleep, the benefits of good quality sleep, and practical tips for improving sleep habits.

Getting adequate sleep is crucial for good health and well-being. During sleep, your body works to repair and restore itself, and your brain processes information and consolidates memories. Lack of sleep can have serious consequences for your physical and mental health, including increased risk for obesity, diabetes, heart disease, and depression.

Most adults need 7-9 hours of sleep per night, while children and teenagers need even more. However, many people fail to get the recommended amount of sleep due to busy schedules, stress, or sleep disorders like insomnia or sleep apnea.

If you struggle with getting enough sleep, there are several strategies you can try to improve your sleep habits. These include creating a consistent sleep schedule, practicing relaxation techniques before bed, avoiding screens and stimulating activities in the evening, and creating a comfortable sleep environment. If you continue to have difficulty sleeping, it's important to talk to your healthcare provider to rule out any underlying medical conditions and explore other treatment options.

Sleep plays a vital role in many aspects of health, including:

1. Physical health: During sleep, your body produces cytokines, which help fight off infection, inflammation, and stress. Lack of sleep can impair your immune system and increase your risk of infections, chronic diseases, and other health problems.

2. Mental health: Sleep is crucial for emotional regulation, mood, and cognitive function. Chronic sleep deprivation can contribute to anxiety, depression, irritability, and difficulty concentrating.

3. Weight management: Sleep plays a role in regulating hormones that control appetite, metabolism, and energy balance. Lack of sleep can disrupt these hormones and increase your risk of weight gain and obesity.

4. Performance and productivity: Sleep is essential for optimal physical and mental performance, including memory, creativity, problem-solving, and decision-making. Lack of sleep can impair these functions and decrease productivity.

Overall, getting enough sleep is a fundamental aspect of a healthy lifestyle. By prioritizing sleep and making changes to improve your sleep habits, you can optimize your physical and mental health and improve your overall well-being.

The Benefits of Good Quality Sleep

This section discusses the many benefits of getting enough good quality sleep, such as improved mood, increased energy, better cognitive function, and a stronger immune system. It also highlights the potential consequences of sleep deprivation, such as increased risk of chronic diseases, impaired judgment, and mood disturbances.

Getting good quality sleep on a regular basis is essential for maintaining good health and well-being. Here are some of the benefits of getting adequate, restful sleep:

1. Improved memory and learning: During sleep, your brain consolidates memories and processes new information, which can improve your ability to learn and retain information.

2. Enhanced mood: Adequate sleep can improve your mood and reduce the risk of mood disorders such as depression and anxiety.

3. Increased productivity: Good quality sleep can improve your energy levels, concentration, and overall cognitive function, which can increase productivity and job performance.

4. Better physical health: Getting enough sleep can help prevent a range of health problems, including obesity, diabetes, heart disease, and stroke. It can also strengthen your immune system, making you less susceptible to illness.

5. Reduced inflammation: Sleep deprivation can cause inflammation throughout the body, which can contribute to a range of health problems. Getting enough sleep can help reduce inflammation and improve overall health.

6. Lowered stress levels: Good quality sleep can help reduce stress levels, leading to improved mental and physical health.

Overall, getting good quality sleep is crucial for maintaining good health and well-being. By prioritizing sleep and making changes to improve your sleep habits, you can enjoy the many benefits of restful, rejuvenating sleep.

Practical Tips for Improving Sleep Habits

This section provides practical advice for improving sleep habits, such as establishing a regular sleep schedule, creating a relaxing sleep environment, avoiding caffeine and alcohol before bedtime, and practicing relaxation techniques. It also covers the importance of avoiding electronic devices before bedtime and getting regular exercise.

If you're struggling with sleep, there are several practical tips you can try to help improve your sleep habits:

1. Stick to a consistent sleep schedule: Try to go to bed and wake up at the same time every day, even on weekends.

2. Create a sleep-conducive environment: Make sure your bedroom is dark, quiet, and cool, and invest in comfortable bedding and pillows.

3. Limit caffeine and alcohol intake: Avoid consuming caffeine or alcohol close to bedtime, as they can interfere with sleep.

4. Relax before bedtime: Develop a relaxing bedtime routine, such as taking a warm bath or practicing relaxation techniques like deep breathing or meditation.

5. Exercise regularly: Regular exercise can help improve sleep quality, but try to avoid exercising too close to bedtime.

6. Avoid screens before bedtime: The blue light emitted by electronic screens can interfere with sleep, so try to avoid using phones, tablets, or computers in the hour leading up to bedtime.

7. Manage stress: Stress and anxiety can make it difficult to sleep, so try to develop healthy stress management habits like exercise, meditation, or therapy.

By incorporating these tips into your daily routine, you can improve your sleep habits and enjoy better sleep on a regular basis. Remember, good quality sleep is essential for maintaining good health and well-being, so it's worth taking the time to prioritize it in your life.

CHAPTER THREE

Stress Management for Better Health

In Chapter 3 of "Fit for Life: A Comprehensive Guide to Health, Fitness, and Dieting", the book explores the important topic of stress management and how it can benefit overall health and well-being. This chapter covers a range of strategies for managing stress, including exercise, hobbies, and social support.

Stress is a natural response to a perceived threat, whether real or imagined. It can come from many sources, including work, relationships, finances, and health issues. While some stress is normal and even beneficial, chronic stress can have negative effects on your mental and physical health. Therefore, it's important to develop healthy strategies for managing stress and improving your overall well-being.

Effects of Chronic Stress

When stress becomes chronic, it can lead to a wide range of negative effects on your health, including:

1. Mental health issues: Chronic stress can lead to anxiety, depression, and other mental health issues.

2. Physical health issues: Chronic stress can increase your risk of developing heart disease, high blood pressure, diabetes, and other chronic health conditions.

3. Digestive problems: Chronic stress can cause digestive issues such as stomach pain, bloating, and constipation.

4. Impaired immune system: Chronic stress can weaken your immune system, making you more susceptible to illness and infection.

5. Sleep problems: Chronic stress can disrupt your sleep, leading to fatigue and decreased cognitive function.

Strategies for Managing Stress

1. Identify the source of your stress: The first step in managing stress is to identify the source of your stress. Once you know what's causing your stress, you can develop a plan for managing it.

2. Practice relaxation techniques: There are many relaxation techniques you can use to manage stress, including deep breathing, meditation, and yoga.

3. Exercise regularly: Exercise is a great way to manage stress, as it can help you relax and improve your mood.

4. Get enough sleep: Getting enough sleep is important for managing stress, as it can help you feel more rested and less irritable.

5. Eat a healthy diet: Eating a healthy diet is important for managing stress, as it can help you feel more energized and focused.

6. Seek support: Talking to friends, family, or a mental health professional can be helpful in managing stress.

7. Manage your time: Learning to manage your time effectively can help you reduce stress and feel more in control of your life.

By incorporating these strategies into your daily routine, you can effectively manage stress and improve your overall health and well-being.

Stress is a normal part of life, but chronic stress can have negative effects on your mental and physical health. Therefore, it's important to develop healthy strategies for managing stress. By identifying the source of your stress, practicing relaxation techniques, exercising regularly, getting enough sleep, eating a healthy diet, seeking support, and managing your time effectively, you can effectively manage stress and improve your overall health and well-being.

Understanding Stress

This section defines stress and explains the different types of stress, including acute stress and chronic stress. It also covers the physical and emotional symptoms of stress and the potential consequences of chronic stress on the body and mind.

Stress is a natural and normal reaction of the human body to perceived threats or challenges. It is a physiological and psychological response that prepares the body to either fight or flee. The body releases stress hormones, such as cortisol and adrenaline, which cause the heart rate and blood pressure to increase, and the muscles to tense up. Stress is not always bad, and in fact, a little bit of stress can be helpful to increase motivation and focus. However, prolonged or chronic stress can have negative effects on the body and mind, leading to physical and mental health problems.

Causes of Stress

Stress can be caused by a variety of factors, including work, relationships, financial issues, health problems, and major life changes such as divorce or the loss of a loved one. Different people may react differently to stressors, and what may be stressful for one person may not be for another. In addition, stress can be acute, such as when dealing with a short-term stressor like a job interview, or chronic, such as when dealing with ongoing stressors like a stressful work environment.

Effects of Stress on the Body

Prolonged or chronic stress can have negative effects on the body. The body's response to stress is designed to be short-term, and when stress is chronic, it can cause the body to stay in a constant state of high alert, which can lead to physical health problems. Some of the physical effects of chronic stress can include:

1. Heart disease: Chronic stress can lead to increased blood pressure, which can increase the risk of heart disease.

2. Digestive problems: Chronic stress can cause digestive problems such as indigestion, stomach ulcers, and irritable bowel syndrome (IBS).

3. Weakened immune system: Chronic stress can weaken the immune system, making the body more susceptible to infections.

4. Sleep problems: Chronic stress can cause sleep problems such as insomnia or frequent waking during the night.

Effects of Stress on the Mind

Stress can also have negative effects on the mind. Chronic stress can lead to mental health problems such as anxiety, depression, and burnout. It can also lead to cognitive problems such as memory loss and difficulty concentrating.

Stress Management Techniques

There are many different techniques that can be used to manage stress. Some of the most effective techniques include:

1. Exercise: Regular exercise can help to reduce stress levels and improve overall physical and mental health.

2. Relaxation techniques: Techniques such as meditation, deep breathing, and yoga can help to reduce stress levels and promote relaxation.

3. Time management: Effective time management can help to reduce stress levels by reducing the feeling of being overwhelmed.

4. Social support: Having a strong social support system can help to reduce stress levels and improve overall mental health.

5. Cognitive-behavioral therapy (CBT): CBT is a type of therapy that can help individuals to identify and change negative thought patterns that contribute to stress.

6. Mindfulness: Mindfulness techniques can help individuals to become more aware of their thoughts and feelings, and to develop a more positive and accepting attitude toward them.

Stress is a normal part of life, but chronic or prolonged stress can have negative effects on both the body and mind. It is important to recognize the signs of stress and to take steps to manage it effectively. By using techniques such as exercise, relaxation techniques, time management, social support, CBT, and mindfulness, individuals can reduce their stress levels and improve their overall physical and mental health.

Exercise and Stress

This section highlights the benefits of exercise for stress management, including reducing stress hormones and promoting the release of endorphins, which can improve mood and reduce anxiety. It provides guidance on how much exercise is needed to achieve these benefits and offers suggestions for types of exercise that can be particularly effective.

Exercise has been shown to be an effective way to manage stress and improve overall mental health. When you exercise, your body releases endorphins, which are natural chemicals that help you feel good and reduce feelings of pain and stress. Exercise also helps reduce the levels of stress hormones in your body, such as cortisol and adrenaline, and helps to lower blood pressure and heart rate.

There are many different types of exercise that can be effective in managing stress, including cardiovascular exercise, strength training, and yoga. Cardiovascular exercise, such as running, cycling, or swimming, can be particularly effective in reducing stress levels. This is because it increases blood flow to the brain, which helps to improve mood and reduce feelings of anxiety.

Strength training is another effective form of exercise for managing stress. Not only does it improve physical health by building muscle mass and reducing the risk of injury, but it can also boost mental health by increasing confidence and self-esteem.

Yoga is a form of exercise that combines physical movements with breathing and meditation. It has been shown to be effective in reducing stress levels, improving mood, and promoting relaxation. In addition, yoga can help improve flexibility, balance, and strength, which can also help reduce the risk of injury.

It's important to remember that exercise should be used as a tool to manage stress, not as a way to add more stress to your life. It's important to find an exercise routine that you enjoy and that fits into your schedule. Start with small, manageable goals and gradually increase the intensity and duration of your exercise as you become more comfortable.

It's also important to listen to your body and to not push yourself too hard. Overexertion can actually increase stress levels and put you at risk of injury. Make sure to take breaks when you need them and to rest and recover between workouts. By incorporating a variety of stress management techniques into your daily routine, you can reduce the negative effects of stress on your body and improve your overall health and well-being.

CHAPTER FOUR

Cardiovascular Exercise for Heart Health

Cardiovascular exercise, also known as aerobic exercise, is any physical activity that increases the heart rate and breathing rate to improve cardiovascular health. Cardiovascular exercise is an essential component of any fitness routine and provides numerous health benefits. In this chapter, we will explore the benefits of cardiovascular exercise, how to incorporate it into your fitness routine, and the best exercises for improving heart health.

Benefits of Cardiovascular Exercise:

1. Improves Heart Health: Cardiovascular exercise strengthens the heart muscle, improves blood flow, and reduces the risk of heart disease.

2. Increases Stamina: Regular cardiovascular exercise improves endurance and increases the body's ability to perform physical activities for extended periods.

3. Aids in Weight Loss: Cardiovascular exercise burns calories and helps create a calorie deficit, leading to weight loss.

4. Reduces Stress and Anxiety: Cardiovascular exercise triggers the release of endorphins, which improve mood and reduce stress and anxiety.

5. Lowers Blood Pressure: Cardiovascular exercise can help lower blood pressure and reduce the risk of hypertension.

Incorporating Cardiovascular Exercise into Your Fitness Routine:

To reap the benefits of cardiovascular exercise, it is recommended to engage in moderate-intensity aerobic exercise for at least 150 minutes per week. You can start with a low-intensity activity, such as walking, and gradually increase the intensity as you build endurance.

Here are some tips for incorporating cardiovascular exercise into your fitness routine:

1. Choose an activity that you enjoy and are more likely to stick to, such as running, cycling, swimming, or dancing.

2. Mix up your routine with different types of cardiovascular exercises to avoid boredom and challenge your body.

3. Start with short sessions of 10-15 minutes and gradually increase the duration and intensity of your workouts.

4. Incorporate cardiovascular exercise into your daily routine by taking the stairs instead of the elevator or walking to work instead of driving.

5. Stay hydrated by drinking plenty of water before, during, and after your workouts.

Best Exercises for Improving Heart Health:

1. Running: Running is an excellent cardiovascular exercise that can improve heart health and endurance.

2. Cycling: Cycling is a low-impact exercise that strengthens the lower body and improves cardiovascular health.

3. Swimming: Swimming is a full-body workout that improves cardiovascular health and is gentle on the joints.

4. High-Intensity Interval Training (HIIT): HIIT workouts involve short bursts of high-intensity exercise followed by rest periods and are effective for improving cardiovascular fitness.

5. Dancing: Dancing is a fun way to get your heart pumping and improve cardiovascular health.

In conclusion, cardiovascular exercise is an essential component of any fitness routine and provides numerous health benefits, including improved heart health, increased stamina, weight loss, stress reduction, and lowered blood pressure. Incorporating cardiovascular exercise into your fitness routine is easy and can be done by choosing an activity you enjoy, gradually increasing intensity and duration, and mixing up your routine with different types of exercises. Remember to stay hydrated and listen to your body to avoid injury.

CHAPTER FIVE

Strength Training for Muscle and Bone Health

This chapter focuses on the importance of muscular strength and endurance for overall health and well-being. It discusses the benefits of strength training, such as increased bone density, improved posture, and reduced risk of injury. It also provides guidance on how to incorporate strength training into a fitness routine, including exercises for different muscle groups and recommendations for frequency and intensity.

Strength training is an essential component of a well-rounded fitness program. It involves performing exercises that challenge your muscles and bones by using resistance, such as weights or resistance bands. While cardiovascular exercise focuses on the heart and lungs, strength training targets the muscles and bones, helping to build strength, improve bone density, and enhance overall health.

One of the primary benefits of strength training is increased muscle mass. As we age, we naturally lose muscle mass, which can lead to weakness, balance issues, and a greater risk of falls. By engaging in regular strength training, we can help maintain and even increase our muscle mass, which can improve our physical function and quality of life.

Another benefit of strength training is increased bone density. Like muscle mass, our bone density naturally decreases as we age, which can lead to osteoporosis and an increased risk of fractures. However, studies have shown that strength training can help increase bone density, reducing the risk of osteoporosis and fractures.

In addition to these physical benefits, strength training has been shown to have a positive impact on mental health as well. Research has found that strength training can help reduce symptoms of depression and anxiety, improve cognitive function, and enhance self-esteem and body image.

When starting a strength training program, it's essential to start slowly and focus on proper form to avoid injury. It's also important to target all major muscle groups, including the legs, back, chest, arms, and core. Aim to do strength training exercises at least two to three times per week, with a day of rest in between sessions to allow your muscles time to recover.

Strength training can be done using free weights, machines, or bodyweight exercises, and there are many resources available to help you create a safe and effective program. Whether you're a beginner or an experienced gym-goer, incorporating strength training into your fitness routine can help improve your physical and mental health and enhance your overall quality of life.

Benefits of Strength Training:

Strength training is beneficial for several reasons, including:

1. Increased Muscle Mass: Strength training increases muscle mass, which can lead to a boost in metabolism and fat loss over time.

2. Increased Bone Density: Strength training places stress on bones, which can stimulate bone growth and increase bone density. This can help reduce the risk of osteoporosis and fractures later in life.

3. Improved Balance and Coordination: Strength training can improve balance and coordination, which can reduce the risk of falls and injuries.

4. Increased Strength and Endurance: As the name suggests, strength training can increase both strength and endurance, allowing you to perform daily tasks with greater ease.

5. Enhanced Mood: Like other forms of exercise, strength training has been shown to improve mood and reduce symptoms of depression and anxiety.

Tips for Effective Strength Training:

Here are some tips to help you get the most out of your strength training routine:

1. Use Proper Form: Proper form is crucial for avoiding injury and getting the most out of your exercises. If you're unsure about proper form, consider working with a personal trainer or fitness professional.

2. Start Slowly: It's important to start with light weights and build up gradually to heavier weights. This can help prevent injury and ensure that you're using proper form.

3. Focus on Compound Exercises: Compound exercises, such as squats, lunges, and deadlifts, work multiple muscle groups at once and are highly effective for building strength.

4. Vary Your Routine: Mixing up your exercises can help prevent boredom and challenge your muscles in new ways. Consider incorporating different types of equipment, such as dumbbells, resistance bands, and kettlebells.

5. Rest and Recover: It's important to give your muscles time to rest and recover between workouts. Aim to strength train 2-3 times per week and give yourself at least one day of rest between sessions.

Overall, strength training is an important component of a well-rounded fitness routine. By incorporating strength training into your workouts, you can improve muscle mass, bone density, balance, and coordination, while also enhancing your overall health and well-being.

CHAPTER SIX

Flexibility and Balance for Injury Prevention

This chapter explores the benefits of flexibility for overall health and well-being, such as improved range of motion, reduced risk of injury, and better posture. It offers suggestions for types of flexibility exercises, such as yoga and stretching, and provides guidance on how to incorporate them into a fitness routine.

Flexibility and balance are two essential components of overall fitness that often get overlooked. They are particularly important for injury prevention, especially as we age. In this chapter, we will discuss the benefits of flexibility and balance, how to improve them, and how to incorporate them into your fitness routine.

The Benefits of Flexibility and Balance

Flexibility refers to the range of motion in your joints and muscles. Maintaining good flexibility is important for several reasons. It helps to prevent injuries by reducing the risk of muscle strains and joint sprains. It also helps to improve posture, which can reduce the risk of back pain and other musculoskeletal issues. Additionally, good flexibility can improve athletic performance by allowing for better range of motion in sports such as gymnastics, dance, and martial arts.

Balance, on the other hand, refers to your ability to maintain your center of gravity over your base of support. Good balance is essential for daily activities such as walking, climbing stairs, and carrying objects. It can also help to reduce the risk of falls, which can be particularly dangerous for older adults.

Improving Flexibility

Improving flexibility can be achieved through a variety of methods. One effective method is through static stretching, which involves holding a stretch for a set period of time. Examples of static stretches include hamstring stretches, quadriceps stretches, and calf stretches. It is important to warm up before performing static stretches to prevent injury.

Another method for improving flexibility is through dynamic stretching, which involves moving your joints through their full range of motion. Examples of dynamic stretches include arm circles, leg swings, and lunges. Dynamic stretching is particularly beneficial before a workout, as it can help to increase blood flow to the muscles and prepare them for exercise.

Yoga is another effective way to improve flexibility. It involves a series of poses that are designed to stretch and strengthen the muscles, as well as improve balance and focus. Many yoga poses also incorporate elements of dynamic stretching, making it an effective way to warm up before exercise.

Improving Balance

Improving balance can also be achieved through a variety of methods. One effective method is through balance exercises, which involve standing on one foot or performing other exercises that challenge your balance. Examples of balance exercises include standing on one foot, walking heel to toe, and performing squats on a balance board.

Another effective way to improve balance is through yoga. Many yoga poses require balance, which can help to improve overall balance and stability. In particular, poses such as Tree Pose and Warrior III require a high level of balance and focus.

Incorporating Flexibility and Balance into Your Fitness Routine

Incorporating flexibility and balance into your fitness routine can be done in a variety of ways. One effective method is to perform a dynamic warm-up before your workout that includes dynamic stretches and balance exercises. This can help to prepare your muscles for exercise and improve overall flexibility and balance.

Another effective way to incorporate flexibility and balance into your routine is through yoga. Yoga classes can be found at most gyms and fitness centers, and many online resources are available as well.

Finally, incorporating flexibility and balance into your daily routine can be as simple as taking a few minutes each day to perform static stretches or balance exercises. This can help to improve overall flexibility and balance, reduce the risk of injury, and improve overall quality of life.

Flexibility refers to the range of motion of your joints and the mobility of your muscles. It is an essential component of physical fitness and plays a crucial role in injury prevention, posture, and balance. Inflexibility can lead to muscle imbalances, which can cause pain, discomfort, and injury. On the other hand, good flexibility can improve your athletic performance, reduce the risk of injury, and enhance your overall quality of life.

There are various ways to improve your flexibility, including stretching exercises, yoga, Pilates, and foam rolling. These activities can help you maintain the elasticity of your muscles and joints, increase blood flow, and reduce muscle tension.

Stretching exercises are the most common way to improve flexibility. They involve elongating your muscles to increase your range of motion gradually. There are two types of stretching exercises: static and dynamic.

Static stretches involve holding a stretch position for a certain amount of time, typically 10 to 30 seconds. Examples of static stretches include hamstring stretches, quad stretches, and calf stretches. These stretches are best done after a workout when your muscles are warm and pliable.

Dynamic stretches, on the other hand, involve moving your muscles through a range of motion. Examples of dynamic stretches include walking lunges, high knees, and butt kicks. These stretches are best done before a workout to prepare your muscles for the activity.

Yoga and Pilates are also excellent ways to improve flexibility. They involve a series of poses that require you to stretch your muscles and hold them in place for an extended period. These activities not only improve flexibility but also promote relaxation, stress reduction, and mental clarity.

Finally, foam rolling is a popular method to improve flexibility and reduce muscle soreness. It involves using a foam roller to apply pressure to different parts of your body to break up adhesions and tightness in your muscles. Foam rolling can be done before or after a workout, or even as a standalone activity.

Overall, improving your flexibility is essential for maintaining good physical health and preventing injury. Incorporating stretching exercises, yoga, Pilates, and foam rolling into your fitness routine can help you improve your flexibility, reduce muscle tension, and enhance your overall well-being.

Flexibility and balance are two essential components of overall fitness that are often overlooked. By incorporating flexibility and balance exercises into your fitness routine, you can reduce the risk of injury, improve athletic performance, and improve overall quality of life. Whether through yoga, static stretching, or balance exercises, there are many ways to improve flexibility and balance and reap the benefits they provide.

CHAPTER SEVEN

The Science of Nutrition

Nutrition is the study of how food affects the body and how the body processes and utilizes the nutrients in food. Good nutrition is essential for maintaining good health, preventing chronic diseases, and promoting overall well-being. In this chapter, we will explore the basics of nutrition, including the six essential nutrients, the digestive system, and the process of metabolism.

The Six Essential Nutrients

There are six essential nutrients that the body needs in order to function properly:

1. Carbohydrates - Carbohydrates are the body's primary source of energy. They are found in foods like bread, pasta, rice, and fruits.

2. Proteins - Proteins are important for building and repairing tissues in the body. They are found in foods like meat, fish, poultry, and beans.

3. Fats - Fats provide energy, help absorb certain vitamins, and protect organs. They are found in foods like butter, oils, nuts, and seeds.

4. Vitamins - Vitamins are essential for a variety of bodily functions, including immune system health, bone growth, and vision. They are found in a wide variety of foods.

5. Minerals - Minerals are important for building strong bones, transmitting nerve impulses, and maintaining a healthy immune system. They are found in foods like milk, cheese, and leafy green vegetables.

6. Water - Water is essential for life and is involved in many bodily processes, including digestion, temperature regulation, and waste removal. It is found in beverages like water, juice, and milk, as well as in fruits and vegetables.

The Digestive System

The digestive system is responsible for breaking down food into nutrients that can be used by the body. It consists of several organs, including the mouth, esophagus, stomach, small intestine, large intestine, rectum, and anus.

The process of digestion begins in the mouth, where food is chewed and mixed with saliva. The food then travels down the esophagus and into the stomach, where it is mixed with stomach acid and digestive enzymes. From there, the food moves into the small intestine, where nutrients are absorbed into the bloodstream. The remaining waste then moves into the large intestine, where water is absorbed and waste products are eliminated.

Metabolism

Metabolism is the process by which the body converts food into energy. It involves two main processes: catabolism and anabolism.

Catabolism is the process of breaking down larger molecules into smaller ones. This process releases energy that can be used by the body.

Anabolism is the process of building larger molecules from smaller ones. This process requires energy.

The rate of metabolism is influenced by several factors, including age, sex, body size, and physical activity level. Eating a healthy diet and getting regular exercise can help to boost metabolism and promote overall health.

Good nutrition is essential for maintaining good health and preventing chronic diseases. By understanding the six essential nutrients, the digestive system, and the process of metabolism, you can make informed choices about the foods you eat and how they affect your body. Eating a well-balanced diet that includes a variety of foods from all food groups is key to promoting overall health and well-being.

CHAPTER EIGHT

Macronutrients and Micronutrients

In this chapter, we will discuss the two categories of nutrients: macronutrients and micronutrients. Understanding the difference between these two categories is important in developing a healthy and balanced diet.

Macronutrients

Macronutrients are nutrients that are required by the body in large amounts. There are three macronutrients: carbohydrates, proteins, and fats.

1. Carbohydrates - Carbohydrates are the body's primary source of energy. They are found in foods like bread, pasta, rice, and fruits. There are two types of carbohydrates: simple and complex. Simple carbohydrates are made up of one or two sugar molecules and are found in foods like candy, soda, and fruit juice. Complex carbohydrates are made up of many sugar molecules and are found in foods like whole grains, fruits, and vegetables.

2. Proteins - Proteins are important for building and repairing tissues in the body. They are found in foods like meat, fish, poultry, and beans. Proteins are made up of amino acids, which are the building blocks of proteins.

3. Fats - Fats provide energy, help absorb certain vitamins, and protect organs. They are found in foods like butter, oils, nuts, and seeds. There are three types of fats: saturated, unsaturated, and trans. Saturated fats are typically found in animal products and can contribute to heart disease. Unsaturated fats are typically found in plant-based foods and can be beneficial for heart health. Trans fats are typically found in processed foods and can contribute to heart disease.

Micronutrients

Micronutrients are nutrients that are required by the body in small amounts. There are two types of micronutrients: vitamins and minerals.

1. Vitamins - Vitamins are essential for a variety of bodily functions, including immune system health, bone growth, and vision. They are found in a wide variety of foods. There are two types of vitamins: water-soluble and fat-soluble. Water-soluble vitamins are not stored in the body and must be consumed regularly. Examples of water-soluble vitamins include vitamin C and the B vitamins. Fat-soluble vitamins are stored in the body and can be toxic in large amounts. Examples of fat-soluble vitamins include vitamins A, D, E, and K.

2. Minerals - Minerals are important for building strong bones, transmitting nerve impulses, and maintaining a healthy immune system. They are found in foods like milk, cheese, and leafy green vegetables. There are two types of minerals: major minerals and

trace minerals. Major minerals are required by the body in larger amounts, while trace minerals are required in smaller amounts. Examples of major minerals include calcium, magnesium, and potassium. Examples of trace minerals include iron, zinc, and copper.

Conclusion

Macronutrients and micronutrients are both essential for maintaining good health. Eating a balanced diet that includes a variety of foods from all food groups can help ensure that you are getting all of the nutrients that your body needs. It is important to pay attention to the types and amounts of macronutrients and micronutrients that you are consuming in order to maintain a healthy and balanced diet.

CHAPTER NINE

Strategies for Healthy Eating

In this chapter, we will discuss some strategies for healthy eating that can help you maintain a balanced diet and achieve your health goals.

1. Plan ahead - Planning your meals and snacks ahead of time can help you make healthier choices and avoid impulsive or unhealthy food choices. Consider planning your meals and snacks for the week and making a grocery list to ensure that you have healthy options available.

2. Choose whole foods - Whole foods, such as fruits, vegetables, whole grains, lean proteins, and healthy fats, provide important nutrients and can help you maintain a healthy weight. Try to choose whole foods over processed foods whenever possible.

3. Practice portion control - Portion control is an important part of maintaining a healthy diet. Pay attention to serving sizes and use measuring cups or a food scale to ensure that you are consuming appropriate portions.

4. Eat mindfully - Mindful eating involves paying attention to the sensory experience of eating, including the taste, smell, and texture of food. This can help you enjoy your food more and eat more slowly, which can lead to better digestion and satisfaction.

5. Stay hydrated - Drinking enough water is important for maintaining good health. Aim to drink at least eight cups of water per day, and more if you are active or in hot weather.

6. Limit processed foods - Processed foods, such as fast food, chips, and sugary snacks, can be high in calories, unhealthy fats, and added sugars. Limiting these foods can help you maintain a healthy weight and reduce your risk of chronic diseases.

7. Practice moderation - It is important to enjoy all foods in moderation, including indulgent treats. Try to find a balance between healthy eating and indulging in your favorite foods.

8. Seek support - Seeking support from friends, family, or a healthcare professional can be helpful in maintaining a healthy diet. Consider joining a cooking class, support group, or working with a registered dietitian to help you achieve your health goals.

Conclusion

Adopting healthy eating habits can have a positive impact on your physical and mental health. By planning ahead, choosing whole foods, practicing portion control, eating mindfully, staying hydrated, limiting processed foods, practicing moderation, and seeking support, you can maintain a balanced diet and achieve your health goals. Remember, small changes can make a big difference, and it is never too late to start making healthier choices.

CHAPTER TEN

Creating a Personalized Health, Fitness, and Diet Plan

In this chapter, we will discuss how to create a personalized health, fitness, and diet plan that is tailored to your individual needs and goals.

Step 1: Define your goals - The first step in creating a personalized plan is to define your health, fitness, and diet goals. What do you want to achieve? Do you want to lose weight, gain muscle, improve your overall health, or all of the above? Be specific and set realistic goals.

Step 2: Assess your current lifestyle - Take a look at your current lifestyle and identify any areas that may be hindering your progress towards your goals. Are you eating too much junk food, not getting enough exercise, or not getting enough sleep? Identify areas where you can make positive changes.

Step 3: Create a plan of action - Based on your goals and current lifestyle, create a plan of action that includes specific actions you will take to achieve your goals. This may include changes to your diet, exercise routine, and sleep habits. Be specific and create measurable goals.

Step 4: Implement your plan - Once you have created your plan of action, it's time to put it into practice. Start with small, achievable goals and gradually work towards bigger goals. Remember that change takes time, so be patient and persistent.

Step 5: Monitor your progress - Regularly monitor your progress towards your goals and make adjustments to your plan as needed. Celebrate your successes and learn from any setbacks.

Step 6: Seek support - Seeking support from friends, family, or a healthcare professional can be helpful in achieving your goals. Consider joining a support group, hiring a personal trainer, or working with a registered dietitian to help you stay on track.

Conclusion

Creating a personalized health, fitness, and diet plan can help you achieve your goals and improve your overall health and well-being. By defining your goals, assessing your current lifestyle, creating a plan of action, implementing your plan, monitoring your progress, and seeking support, you can create a plan that is tailored to your individual needs and goals. Remember to be patient, persistent, and flexible, and celebrate your successes along the way.

CHAPTER ELEVEN

Staying Motivated and Overcoming Obstacles

Staying motivated and overcoming obstacles is a critical component of achieving any health, fitness, or diet goals. In this section, we will discuss some tips for staying motivated and overcoming obstacles.

1. Set achievable goals - Setting realistic and achievable goals is essential to staying motivated. Start with small, measurable goals, and gradually work your way up to more challenging goals.

2. Find your why - Identify your reasons for wanting to achieve your health, fitness, or diet goals. Whether it's improving your health, boosting your confidence, or setting a good example for your family, having a clear why can help you stay motivated when faced with challenges.

3. Use positive self-talk - The way you talk to yourself can have a big impact on your motivation. Use positive self-talk to reinforce your goals and remind yourself of your why.

4. Create a support network - Having a support network of friends, family, or professionals can help you stay motivated and overcome obstacles. Consider joining a support group, working with a personal trainer, or hiring a registered dietitian to help you stay on track.

5. Reward yourself - Set up a system of rewards for achieving your goals. This can be as simple as treating yourself to a movie or a new workout outfit, or something more significant like a vacation or a spa day.

6. Embrace setbacks - Setbacks are a normal part of any journey towards health and wellness. Instead of getting discouraged, use setbacks as an opportunity to learn and grow.

7. Stay flexible - Being flexible with your goals and plans can help you overcome obstacles and stay motivated. If you are facing a challenge, try to find a new approach that works for you.

Conclusion

Staying motivated and overcoming obstacles is key to achieving any health, fitness, or diet goals. By setting achievable goals, finding your why, using positive self-talk, creating a support network, rewarding yourself, embracing setbacks, and staying flexible, you can stay motivated and overcome obstacles on your journey towards better health and wellness. Remember that change takes time, and be patient and persistent in your efforts.

CHAPTER TWELVE

Maintaining Your Health and Wellness Long-Term

Maintaining your health and wellness long-term is essential for achieving lasting results. In this section, we will discuss some tips for maintaining your health and wellness long-term.

1. Make it a lifestyle - Instead of treating healthy habits as a temporary fix, make them a permanent part of your lifestyle. This means making sustainable changes to your diet, exercise routine, and sleep habits that you can maintain over the long-term.

2. Be consistent - Consistency is key when it comes to maintaining your health and wellness long-term. Make healthy habits a daily part of your routine, and stick to them even when life gets busy or stressful.

3. Find activities you enjoy - Exercise and physical activity should be enjoyable, not a chore. Find activities you enjoy, whether it's hiking, dancing, or playing a team sport, and incorporate them into your routine.

4. Practice mindfulness - Practicing mindfulness, such as meditation or yoga, can help you stay focused and present in the moment. This can help you make better decisions about your health and wellness and stay motivated over the long-term.

5. Stay accountable - Having accountability can help you stay on track with your health and wellness goals. Consider working with a personal trainer, joining a fitness class, or partnering with a friend or family member who shares your goals.

6. Continuously educate yourself - Stay informed about the latest research and best practices in health and wellness. This can help you make informed decisions about your health and wellness and stay motivated over the long-term.

Conclusion

Maintaining your health and wellness long-term is essential for achieving lasting results. By making healthy habits a permanent part of your lifestyle, being consistent, finding activities you enjoy, practicing mindfulness, staying accountable, and continuously educating yourself, you can maintain your health and wellness over the long-term. Remember that change takes time, and be patient and persistent in your efforts.

Conclusion

Your Journey to Health and Fitness Starts Now!

Congratulations! You have taken the first step towards improving your health and fitness by reading this guide. Remember that your journey towards better health and fitness is a process that takes time and effort, but the benefits are well worth it. By following the tips and strategies outlined in this guide, you can create a personalized plan that works for you and achieve your health and fitness goals.

Remember to set realistic goals, find activities you enjoy, be consistent, and stay motivated. Don't be discouraged by setbacks, as they are a normal part of the process. Use them as an opportunity to learn and grow, and stay focused on your why.

Finally, remember that health and wellness is a lifelong journey, and maintaining your health and fitness long-term is key to achieving lasting results. Make healthy habits a permanent part of your lifestyle, stay accountable, and continuously educate yourself.

Your journey to health and fitness starts now. Good luck, and best wishes for a healthier, happier you!